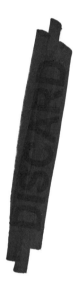

The Library of Sexual Health™

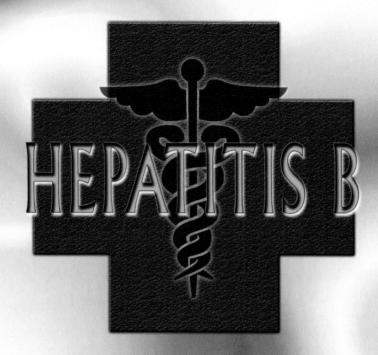

HEPATITIS B

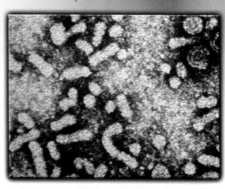

JERI FREEDMAN

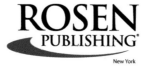
ROSEN
PUBLISHING®
New York

To my niece and nephew, Matthew and Laura Freedman, with love

Published in 2009 by The Rosen Publishing Group, Inc.
29 East 21st Street, New York, NY 10010

Library of Congress Cataloging-in-Publication Data

Freedman, Jeri.
Hepatitis B / Jeri Freedman.—1st ed.
    p. cm.—(the library of sexual health)
Includes bibliographical references.
ISBN-13: 978-1-4358-5058-3 (library binding)
1. Hepatitis B—Popular works. I. Title.
RC848.H44F74 2009
616.3'623—dc22

2008006852

Manufactured in Malaysia

CONTENTS

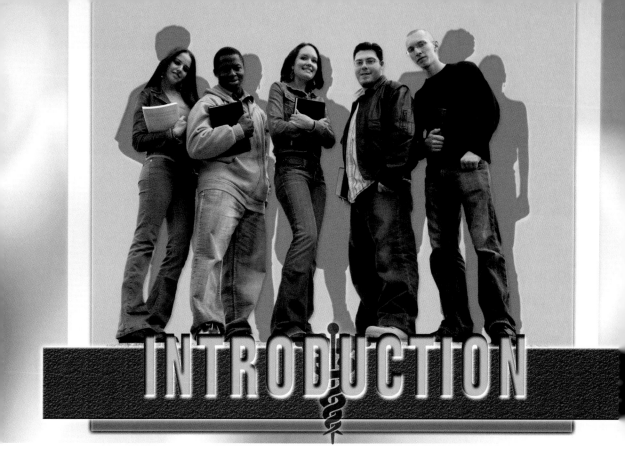

INTRODUCTION

H epatitis is a disease of the liver. *Hepa* comes from the Greek word for liver, and *itis* is Latin for "inflammation." Thus, hepatitis is "inflammation of the liver." When you have hepatitis, your liver doesn't work normally. In rare cases, the liver can fail altogether. Your liver plays a key role in keeping you healthy, purifying your blood, and supplying chemicals that your body needs. Liver disease can have serious short- and long-term effects on your health.

Hepatitis is not a single disease. Rather, it is inflammation of the liver that can result from various causes. Most forms of hepatitis come from infection with a virus. There are different types of hepatitis viruses, including hepatitis A, B, C, D, E, and G. This book deals specifically with hepatitis B. Hepatitis B is carried in the blood and other body fluids and is caused by the hepatitis B virus (HBV). It is most often passed from one person to another in semen or blood as a result of having unprotected sex or from sharing a hypodermic needle. It may also be contracted from blood transfusions, although this is rare. It is also possible to pass on HBV via saliva, tears, or sweat, if

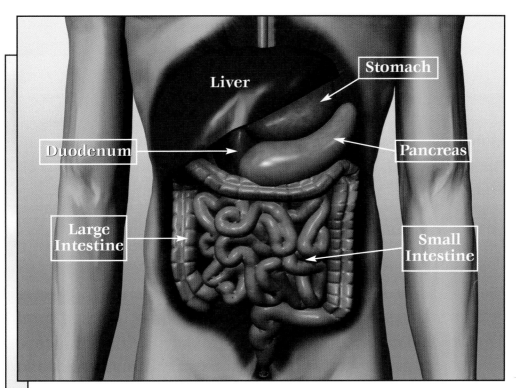

The liver is located in the upper-right portion of the abdominal cavity. It is the largest internal organ.

there is direct contact with a cut or scratch. However, this type of transmission is less likely because the concentration of the virus is lower in these fluids.

This book starts out by explaining how the liver functions, how hepatitis infects the liver and affects its function, and how you might contract hepatitis. It then goes on to discuss the short- and long-term effects of hepatitis, its diagnosis and treatment, and ways you can protect yourself so that you reduce your chances of catching it.

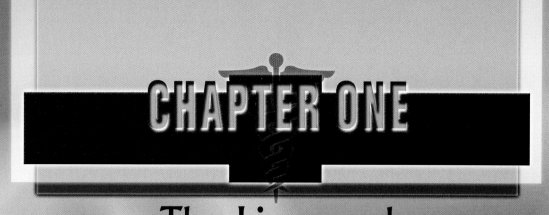

CHAPTER ONE

The Liver and Hepatitis B

The liver is a reddish-brown organ located beneath the right side of your rib cage, beside the stomach. Your liver is your largest gland. (A gland produces chemicals that affect various processes in the body.) Your liver is also your second-largest organ, after your skin.

The liver is composed of two lobes, right and left. Large blood vessels connect the liver to the stomach, pancreas, spleen, and small intestine. This allows blood from these organs to flow into the liver, where the blood's nutrients are processed.

Much of the liver is structured like a large sieve. Blood from the organs travels from large blood vessels into a series of smaller blood vessels called capillaries. The capillaries contain many small openings called pores. These allow blood to pass to and from the liver cells, which are called hepatocytes (*cyte* means "cell"). The liver is one of the few organs in the body that can regenerate, or grow back, when a piece is removed.

FUNCTIONS OF THE LIVER

Your liver performs many vital functions. It cleans toxins and chemicals out of your blood so that they do not build up to harmful levels. It stores glycogen, a form of sugar that the body burns for energy. It produces proteins that allow your blood to clot when you are injured. It produces enzymes, which are chemicals necessary for bodily processes such as digestion. Your liver also breaks down red blood cells when they age.

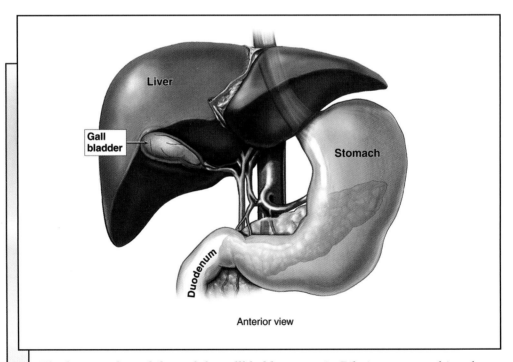

Anterior view

The liver produces bile, and the gallbladder stores it. Bile is transported in tubes called bile ducts. The duodenum is the first part of the small intestine, which connects to the stomach.

One of the primary functions of the liver is to regulate how much cholesterol there is in your body. Cholesterol is a fatty substance that the body uses to produce hormones—chemicals that control bodily functions. In addition to the cholesterol produced in the liver, we also get cholesterol from the fat in food that we eat. When too much cholesterol is present in the bloodstream, it can stick to the walls of blood vessels and clog them. When this happens, it can lead to heart attacks and strokes.

Another function of the liver is to produce bile, a liquid necessary for good digestion. Some of the bile goes directly into the intestines, where it helps break down the fat we eat. Excess bile is stored in the gallbladder, an organ located on the underside of the liver.

The liver also breaks down many different medications so that they can be removed from the body. This prevents chemicals from building up in your body and harming you. In addition, it stores a variety of substances that your body needs to function correctly, including vitamin B12, copper, and iron.

WHAT HAPPENS IF THE LIVER FAILS?

As you can see, the liver performs many functions that are critical to keeping you healthy. If the liver becomes damaged or fails altogether, the effects are serious. When the liver fails, it affects your entire body. Toxins may build up in your blood, damaging other organs. Your muscles may waste away due to a lack of proteins to build them up. Your body may have problems regulating the hormones that affect various bodily processes. You may also suffer from mental confusion due to the buildup of the chemical ammonia in the brain. It is very important to keep your liver healthy and disease-free.

HOW DOES HEPATITIS B AFFECT THE BODY?

Hepatitis B can affect the body in many ways. When the liver is diseased, the ducts, or tubes through which the bile passes into the digestive tract, may become blocked, leading to problems in digesting fatty foods. In addition, liver disease affects the balance of cholesterol in the body. Since the liver is involved in eliminating excess cholesterol from the body, a diseased liver may allow excess cholesterol to build up in the body, clogging the arteries.

Cholesterol is needed to manufacture certain hormones in the adrenal glands and in the testes and ovaries, including the male hormone testosterone and the female hormone estrogen. These hormones control the development of normal male and female sex characteristics. When the liver is diseased, problems with the sex hormones may result. For instance, males may develop female characteristics such as enlarged breasts.

Cholesterol is also used to produce thyroid hormones. The thyroid is a butterfly-shaped gland located in the throat. It produces hormones that regulate such basic bodily functions as the production of cells and the generation of energy from fat and sugar. Liver disease can also affect the liver's ability to produce important blood-clotting proteins. These proteins are necessary to stop an injured blood vessel from bleeding.

People with hepatitis B often feel tired. One reason for this is that the liver is a key site for the storage of a type of sugar called glucose, which your body burns for fuel. Your liver stores glucose in a form called glycogen. When necessary, it breaks down glycogen into glucose and releases the glucose into your bloodstream, where it

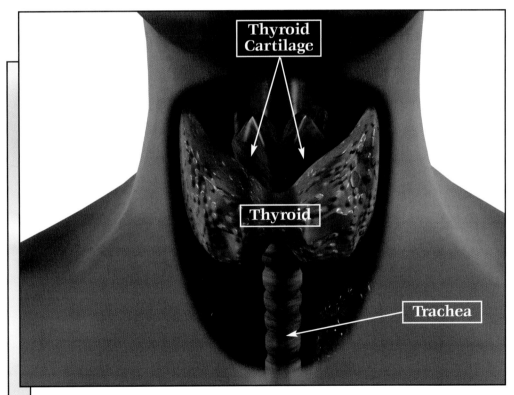

The thyroid gland uses cholesterol in the blood to produce hormones that control cellular processes throughout the body. The trachea is also called the windpipe.

is carried to the cells throughout your body. In the cells, it is "burned" with oxygen to produce energy. When the liver is diseased, it doesn't adequately control the storage and release of glucose, and this leads to fatigue. As you can see, hepatitis B can have serious effects on your whole body.

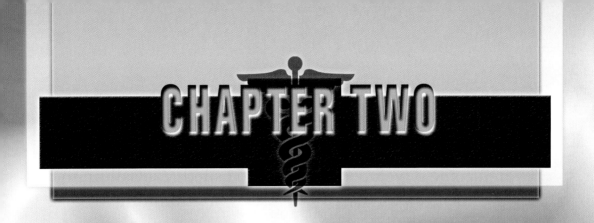

CHAPTER TWO

The Nature of Hepatitis B

T his chapter begins with a look at discoveries related to hepatitis B. It then provides some information on how you might get hepatitis B, what its symptoms are, and what its long-term effects are.

THE HISTORY OF HEPATITIS

Hepatitis is a disease that has been known since ancient times. References to infectious hepatitis epidemics (the rapid spread of a disease to large numbers of people) date back to 2000 BCE. The disease is known to have existed among the Incan, Aztec, and Mayan cultures in the Americas. In medieval times, a Spanish doctor named Moses Maimonides (1113–1204) described hepatitis in his writings.

It has been obvious since ancient times that viral hepatitis is contagious, meaning it can spread from person to person. However, no one knew how it spread until the 1940s. At that time, British doctor F. O. MacCallum was responsible for developing a vaccine to keep soldiers in

Africa from getting a disease called yellow fever. He noticed that many of the soldiers injected with the yellow fever vaccine developed hepatitis. This led MacCallum to suspect that hepatitis might be transmitted in human blood. He thought the virus that caused hepatitis was being spread in the specks of blood left on the needles he reused to vaccinate multiple soldiers. (The needles were not sterilized between injections.) In 1947, MacCallum identified two different strains of hepatitis viruses: A and B. Hepatitis A is generally spread by eating or drinking contaminated food and water. Hepatitis B is spread by contact with bodily fluids.

In 1963, American doctors Baruch Blumberg and Harvey Alter discovered an antigen in the blood of people who had been infected with hepatitis B. (An antigen is a foreign particle that sets off a reaction in a person's immune system.) It was called the "Australian antigen" because it was found in the blood of Australian aborigines, or natives. In this case, the antigen was a component of the outer shell of the hepatitis B virus. This antigen is now referred to as HBsAg (hepatitis B surface antigen). In the late 1960s, Blumberg and his colleagues established that HBsAg is a key component of the hepatitis B virus, and the antigen is now the basis of the hepatitis B vaccine.

In 1970, a British doctor, D. S. Dane, viewed and described entire hepatitis B viruses in blood samples. He used an electron microscope, an extremely powerful tool that allows one to observe particles too small to see with a

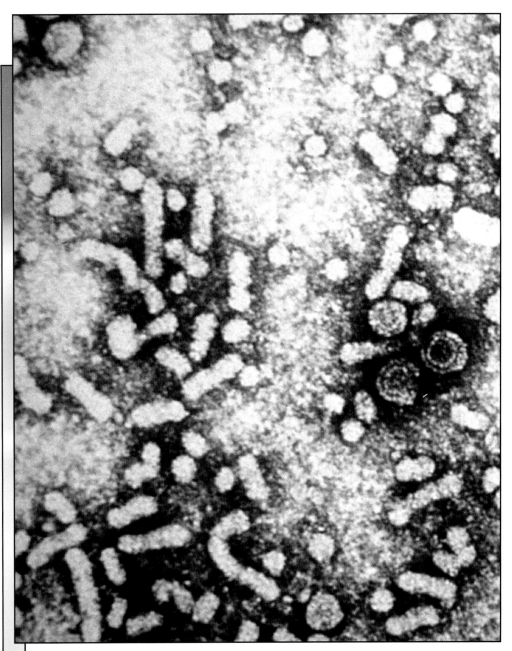

This electron microscope picture shows hepatitis B viruses in a cell. The round spheres are whole viruses; the rod-like shapes are from the outer shell of the virus.

standard microscope. In 1975, Wolf Szmuness, Maurice Hilleman, and their colleagues began testing a hepatitis B vaccine. By 1981, a hepatitis B vaccine made from blood serum (the clear part of blood in which blood cells float) was approved for use.

In the 1980s, William Rutter, an American scientist who founded the biotechnology company Chiron, created the first genetically engineered vaccine for hepatitis B. This vaccine was produced in yeast cells and did not require using human blood, so it was safer from contamination. In 1986, this vaccine was approved by the U.S. Food and Drug Administration (FDA) for use by the general public. In the late twentieth century and early twenty-first century, advances in biotechnology paved the way for new treatments for hepatitis B. These will be discussed in chapter 4.

WHAT CAUSES HEPATITIS B?

Hepatitis B is caused by a virus, a tiny organism that consists of a core of DNA (deoxyribonucleic acid) surrounded by a protective shell. The DNA carries the genetic code for reproducing copies of the virus. The hepatitis B virus attaches itself to the membrane that surrounds a liver cell and injects its DNA core into the cell. The virus takes over the cell and causes it to reproduce the virus's DNA instead of the cell's DNA. When the liver cell is filled with copies of the virus, it bursts. The virus then spreads to nearby cells, and the process is repeated. In this way, the virus can cause widespread damage by destroying the liver's cells.

HOW DO YOU GET HEPATITIS B?

You can get hepatitis B when the virus carried in the blood or semen of another person is transferred into your bloodstream through direct contact. From there, it travels to the liver and infects the cells there. The two common ways of getting hepatitis B are by sharing needles and by having

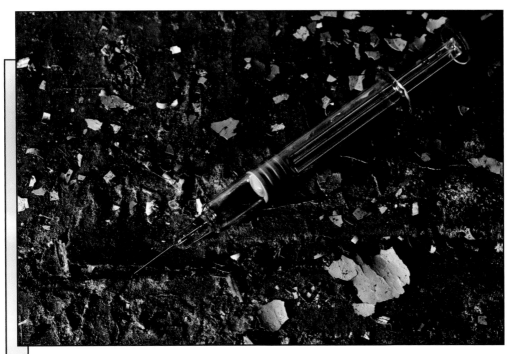

When an infected person injects a drug, a little blood flows back into the needle. This blood is then injected into the next person who uses it, spreading the disease.

unprotected sex. In the case of illegal drug use, users get it by sharing a needle with someone who has the disease. Needles used in tattooing and body piercing can also spread the disease if they are not properly sterilized.

Having unprotected sex means that if your partner is infected, the hepatitis B virus in that person's semen or other bodily fluids can enter your body through any break in your skin.

Hepatitis B may also be contracted from a blood transfusion with infected blood. However, screening is so thorough today at blood banks in the United States and Canada that this is rare.

WHAT ARE THE SYMPTOMS OF HEPATITIS B?

Generally, the symptoms of hepatitis B occur six to fifteen weeks after exposure to the virus. The most common symptoms indicate that the liver is not performing its necessary functions. For example, one of the most obvious symptoms of the disease is jaundice, a yellowing of the skin and eyes. When the liver breaks down red blood cells, it uses some of the resulting components to produce a substance called bilirubin. Bilirubin is one of the elements the liver uses to make bile, a chemical used in digestion. When the liver becomes diseased, it doesn't process bilirubin as well, so excess bilirubin builds up in the blood. Because bilirubin is yellow, this excess bilirubin in the blood makes the skin and eyes look yellow.

Many people naturally have a yellowish tinge to their skin, so looking at skin color is not always a good way to judge whether someone is jaundiced. Looking at the whites of the eyes may be more helpful. These are normally white in everybody, so yellow eyes are a more telling sign of jaundice. Measuring bilirubin in the blood is the most accurate way to know.

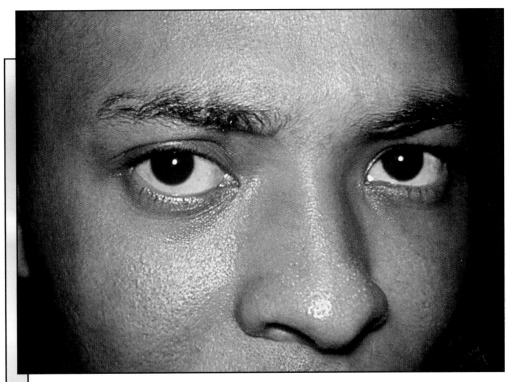

This patient shows symptoms of jaundice from hepatitis. The whites of his eyes and the skin on his face are yellow.

Another major symptom of hepatitis B is fatigue, or a lack of energy. People with hepatitis may also experience flu-like symptoms, including fever and joint pain, nausea, and vomiting. Because excess bilirubin is excreted into urine, dark urine is another sign of possible hepatitis. One may also have pain in the upper-right part of the abdomen.

Many cases of hepatitis resolve, or clear up, on their own. If hepatitis doesn't clear up and the virus remains in your system for a long time, this is called chronic hepatitis. Usually, hepatitis is considered chronic if it lasts for more than six months. About 5 percent of people infected with hepatitis B develop chronic hepatitis, which can damage the liver. Severe liver damage can result in bloating and unexplained weight gain. It can also lead to intense itching. Another sign of a severely affected liver is mental confusion and difficulty in remembering simple things. This is the result of inflammation in the membranes that cover the brain caused by the buildup of ammonia, which is normally broken down by the liver.

THE LONG-TERM EFFECTS OF HEPATITIS B

When hepatitis B continues for a long time, permanent liver damage can occur. One type of damage is cirrhosis. In cirrhosis, normal liver cells die and are replaced with scar tissue. The scar tissue can keep blood from flowing normally through the liver. Then the liver cannot perform its function of filtering blood, and the scarring may

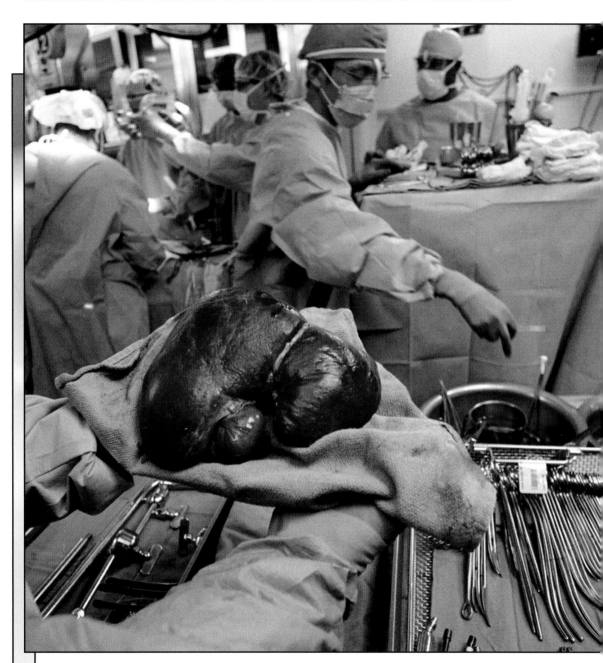

Above is a diseased liver that was removed by doctors. The patient will receive a healthy liver taken from the body of a donor who has recently died.

interfere with the liver's ability to get necessary substances into the blood. Cirrhosis is caused by many types of liver disease, not just hepatitis, but it is one of the problems that hepatitis can lead to. Mild-to-moderate cirrhosis can be treated, so it is not necessarily fatal, especially if it is caught early.

It is known that chronic hepatitis B can lead to liver cancer, although exactly how this happens is not known. Some scientists point to the changes made to a cell's DNA when the virus takes over liver cells and inserts its own DNA. It's possible that in the process, the virus sometimes removes the part of the cell's DNA that regulates reproduction. The liver cells then start multiplying uncontrollably. Liver cancer is one of the few cancers that is increasing, rather than decreasing in the United States, a trend that may be due to an increase in the number of people with chronic hepatitis.

If cirrhosis goes unchecked, the liver can fail. This means that so many liver cells have died, the organ can no longer function. When the liver fails, toxins such as ammonia are not removed from the body and may build up in the organs, including the brain. Ultimately, this may lead to swelling in the brain, coma (unconsciousness), and even death. Toxin buildup may also lead to failure of the lungs and kidneys. If the liver fails completely, often the only hope for the patient is a liver transplant. Chapter 4 provides more information on transplants.

HEPATITIS AND SEXUAL HEALTH

If you contract chronic hepatitis, you will have to tell your partner that you have the disease prior to having sex. You will also have to take precautions not to pass it along. If you are a male with chronic hepatitis and you want to father a child, you face the difficult issue of having unprotected sex with your partner. By doing this, you risk infecting your partner with your disease. What's worse, if the mother is infected, there is a good chance that the baby will be infected as well.

If you are a female who has chronic hepatitis, it may be passed along to the baby through contact with your blood when the baby is born. It may also be passed along when your blood circulates between you and your child through the umbilical cord. About 90 percent of babies infected in this way develop chronic hepatitis, which affects them for their entire lives. If a mother has chronic hepatitis B, immunizing her baby shortly after birth can reduce transmission of the virus.

In general, it is really important to protect yourself against hepatitis B for your own sake, for the sake of any partner you may have in the future, and for the sake of any children you may have.

Ten Facts About Hepatitis B

1. Hepatitis means "inflammation of the liver."

2. An estimated 400 million people worldwide have chronic hepatitis B.

3. About 1.25 million people in the United States have chronic hepatitis B.

4. About 30 percent of people infected with the hepatitis B virus show no symptoms.

5. About 5,000 people in the United States die of hepatitis-related disease annually.

6. In Canada, 250,000 people have chronic hepatitis, according to the Ontario Service Safety Alliance.

7. Young children (newborns to four years of age) who become infected with HBV are the most likely to develop chronic infection.

8. Death from chronic liver disease occurs in 15–25 percent of people with chronic hepatitis B infection.

9. Hepatitis B vaccine is available for all age groups to prevent hepatitis B virus infection.

10. In the last twenty-five years, the greatest decline in new hepatitis B infections has occurred among children and adolescents due to routine vaccination.

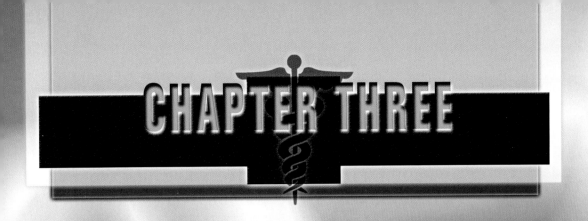

CHAPTER THREE

Preventing Hepatitis B

As mentioned in the preceding chapter, you can get hepatitis B in several ways. However, the most common way is through sexual contact. For this reason, when you are ready to be sexually active, it is important that you take steps to protect yourself.

PUTTING YOURSELF AT RISK

Having unprotected sex can put you at risk for contracting hepatitis B, as well as other sexually transmitted diseases such as HIV, syphilis, gonorrhea, and chlamydia. Therefore, when you decide to have sex, make sure that you use latex condoms. Also, the more sexual partners you have, the greater your likelihood is of getting infected. Your sexual health relies on your good judgment. Avoid using recreational drugs and alcohol, which affect your judgment and therefore lead to risky behavior.

Hepatitis B is a worldwide problem. In the United States, widespread vaccination of children is helping increase immunity to the disease. (See more about this in the next chapter.) Because the vaccine is expensive, however, people in many parts of the world, especially developing countries, are not vaccinated against the disease. So, regardless of where you are, you can't assume that a potential partner has been vaccinated.

The hepatitis B virus is more likely to be transmitted between male partners. However, hepatitis B can easily be transmitted during intercourse between a man and a woman, so women need to take precautions as well. If you find yourself attracted to someone with hepatitis B, you should be vaccinated. You should also be careful about coming in contact with items that might contain the other person's blood, like razors or toothbrushes.

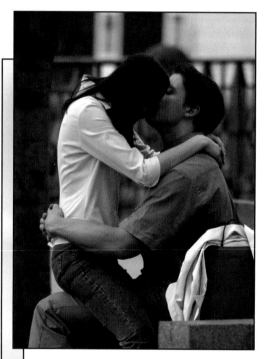

It's important to ask about the health status of your romantic partners. If you don't, it could affect your health as well as the health of your future partners.

RESISTING PRESSURE

As with any important move that you make in life, decision-making and communication skills are important in deciding whether to have sex with another person and in deciding how to do so in a safe way. Don't be pressured into having sex before you're ready. How do you know if you're ready? If you feel nervous and uncertain when the subject comes up, you may not be ready. You shouldn't have sex to seem cool or to fit in with a trendy crowd. You should not agree to have sex with someone because you are embarrassed to say no, because he or she might reject you, or because people might think you're a nerd. If someone cares about you, he or she should care about more than just having sex.

Don't believe everything your friends or schoolmates claim they've done. People like to sound as if they're popular and experienced. Many people exaggerate their sexual experience in order to impress their friends. Don't agree to have sex because you think "everyone else is doing it." In reality, the trend among teenagers is to wait longer before having sex because of the dangers of sexually transmitted diseases. Contrary to the image of teenagers portrayed in movies and popular television shows, everyone is not constantly sleeping with everyone else. Reality TV shows featuring rich young people give a particularly distorted view of the lives of young people. A 2006 study by the Guttmacher Institute reveals that teenagers are waiting longer to start having sex and that 75 percent of teen girls have their first sexual encounter with a steady boyfriend, fiancé, or someone they are married to or living with.

If you don't feel that you are ready to have sex, spend some time thinking about what you'll say if you are asked to, or role-play with a friend so that you are prepared when the subject comes up. Don't abuse drugs or alcohol, which cloud your judgment. If you are in doubt about whether or not to have sex, err on the side of caution. As an added precaution, many people use the buddy system. Go to clubs and parties with a friend, and agree that you will stop each other from doing something you may later regret.

Myths and Facts

MYTH: Hepatitis B is rare, so I'm not likely to come into contact with someone who has it.
FACT: Hepatitis B is one of the most common contagious diseases in the world today. Most studies estimate that between 300 million and 500 million people worldwide are infected with the hepatitis B virus.

MYTH: If a person doesn't have any symptoms of hepatitis B, then I don't have to worry about having sex with him or her.
FACT: About a third of people who are infected with the hepatitis B virus don't experience any symptoms and may not even know that they have the disease. These people can still pass the virus on to someone else, however.

MYTH: If I catch hepatitis B, I can take the hepatitis B vaccine at that time to cure it.
FACT: The vaccine only protects you against the virus if you are vaccinated with it before you come in contact with the virus.

MYTH: I can get hepatitis B only if I have vaginal intercourse.
FACT: You can get hepatitis B from any type of sexual contact. The U.S. Centers for Disease Control and Prevention (CDC) recommends using a latex condom, but the exact effectiveness against hepatitis B is not known. The best protection is immunization.

CHAPTER FOUR

Diagnosing and Treating Hepatitis B

Preventing a problem beforehand is better than having to solve it later. There are ways that you can protect yourself against hepatitis B. One way is to get vaccinated against the disease.

VACCINATION AND IMMUNITY

When a person has hepatitis B, his or her immune system generates antibodies to the virus. Antibodies are proteins that attach themselves to foreign particles so that other immune system cells can recognize and destroy those particles. The body makes a different antibody for each type of bacteria, toxin, or virus that gets into the body. Once antibodies against a particular foreign particle are created, your body continues to produce them. Therefore, once you've had hepatitis B, the antibodies in your system will recognize and attach themselves to the virus if you come in contact with it again. Then your immune system cells will destroy it. This resistance to infection is called immunity.

There is another way to achieve immunity, however: vaccination. When you are vaccinated, you are injected with a small amount of fluid that contains components of the virus. This causes your body to produce specific antibodies to the virus. However, because you are not injected with a functioning form of the virus, you do not get sick. In most cases, vaccination makes you immune to the virus so that if you are later exposed, you do not get the disease.

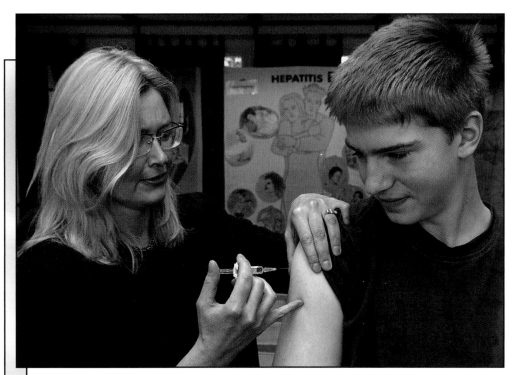

For hepatitis B vaccination, a doctor or nurse injects you with protein from the hepatitis B virus. Vaccination is the surest way to protect yourself.

Today, most hepatitis B vaccines are made by using protein from hepatitis B viruses grown in yeast cells. When the solution containing the hepatitis B protein is injected, the person's body in most cases starts making antibodies for it. These antibodies will then recognize and attach themselves to the actual hepatitis B particles, which contain the same protein. Some years ago, the U.S. and Canadian governments began recommending that all children be given vaccinations for hepatitis B. These vaccinations have been successful in reducing the number of new cases of hepatitis. Recently the U.S. Centers for Disease Control and Prevention (CDC) has been encouraging adults who are not vaccinated to get vaccinations as well. This is especially true for teenagers who were not vaccinated as children. According to the Guttmacher Institute, "although 15–24-year-olds represent only one-quarter of the sexually active population, they account for nearly half of all new STIs [sexually transmitted infections] each year."

DETECTING AND DIAGNOSING HEPATITIS

As with most diseases, the sooner you find out that you have hepatitis B, the better. This is especially true if you have chronic hepatitis. Numerous medications are now available to treat this disease, and the sooner it is caught, the less damage it will do to your liver. For this reason, you should have regular checkups with your doctor and let the doctor know immediately if you have any symptoms.

Various tools are used to diagnose hepatitis. First, a doctor will get your medical history. He or she will ask you questions about your symptoms, your family health history, and your past behavior. Next, the doctor will give you a physical examination. The doctor will look for jaundice, which is an obvious sign of liver disease, but he or she will look for other signs as well. If your weight is too high or too low, this may be a sign of a liver problem.

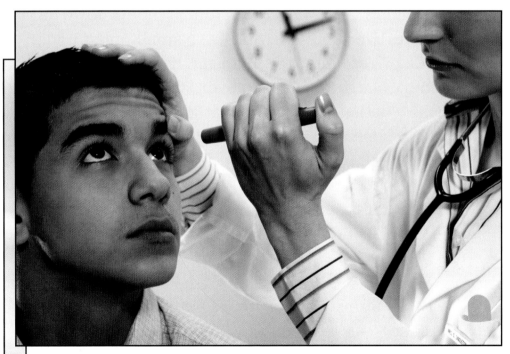

Even though you feel healthy, it's important to have regular checkups with your doctor. Doctors are trained to spot symptoms of disease you might not notice.

Your doctor will also look for signs of liver disease that affect the skin. For example, liver disease can make the skin of the palms of the hands look red. Irregular bruising, too, can be a sign of liver trouble. This is because a diseased liver does not produce an adequate amount of clotting proteins. So, people with hepatitis are more likely to keep bleeding internally from injuries to blood vessels when they bump into things, producing a bruise.

People with chronic liver disease may have red spots with tiny lines coming off them on their arms, shoulders, and chest. These spots are called spider angiomata, or sometimes just "spiders." (*Angio* refers to blood vessels, which are where the spots come from.) The doctor will also feel your liver and your spleen, a small organ under the left side of your rib cage. Both the liver and spleen can become enlarged when the liver is diseased. If the doctor suspects that you have hepatitis after examining you, you may need to undergo testing.

TESTS FOR HEPATITIS

Several different types of tests can reveal if a person has hepatitis. This section explains the different types.

Blood Tests for Hepatitis

Blood tests are important for finding out if a person has hepatitis. They can also be used to monitor how the liver is working and to see if the hepatitis is getting better or worse. In addition, blood tests tell whether the level of liver enzymes is normal or abnormal.

A basic type of blood test is the complete blood count (CBC), which measures how many red blood cells, white blood cells, and platelets you have. If you have liver disease, you may have an abnormally low number of red blood cells, the cells that carry oxygen throughout the body. Even more significant is the platelet count. Platelets are small blood cells produced in the spleen. They help blood to clot. When the liver becomes diseased, blood flow from the spleen to the liver may be blocked. The spleen then swells, trapping the platelets in it. As a result, the number of platelets circulating in the blood decreases, leading to an increase in bleeding and bruising problems.

Certain blood-clotting tests called the prothrombin time (PT) and partial prothromboplastin time (PTT) can reveal liver problems. These tests measure how long it takes your blood to clot. Factors that make blood clot are produced in your liver, so if it takes an abnormally long time for your blood to clot, you may have liver disease.

Blood can also be analyzed to see if it contains hepatitis B antigens. These are proteins that form part of the shell of the hepatitis B virus.

Enzymes are chemicals that speed up processes in the body. Two enzyme tests look for alanine aminotransferase (ALT), which is present in liver cells, and aspartate aminotransferase, which is also found in muscle and heart cells.

High levels of these enzymes in your blood mean that these cells are dying and breaking down. Albumin is a protein made in the liver. When the liver doesn't work right, it doesn't make enough albumin. A blood test will show if the level of albumin in the blood is too low. Finally, the amount of ammonia in the blood can be measured. Too much ammonia in the blood is a sign of liver disease.

Liver Scanning

Doctors can use medical technology to take a closer look at the liver. Techniques include:

- **Ultrasound.** In this test, the technician moves a device that emits sound waves over the liver. A computer analyzes the waves as they bounce off the organ and create a picture of the liver.
- **Magnetic resonance imaging (MRI).** In this test, the patient is placed in a machine that contains large magnets. When the magnets are turned on, they create a magnetic field that causes all of the hydrogen atoms in the body to line up. Radio waves are then bounced off the atoms, causing them to spin. As the waves move, they give off an electrical signal. A computer measures the strength of the resulting signal in different areas and creates a picture of the liver.

- **CAT scan.** Computerized axial tomography (CAT) scans create an image of the liver by bouncing low-radiation X-rays off it at various angles, while the patient lies inside a doughnut-shaped scanner.

Liver Biopsy

A liver biopsy is an invasive way to look at a small piece of the liver. It can tell doctors things that mere images of

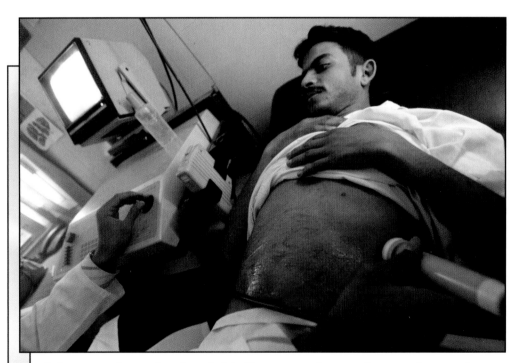

A doctor at a hepatology hospital in Egypt uses ultrasound to examine a patient. Hepatology is the field of study concerned with the liver.

the liver cannot. Since it requires removing a small piece of the liver, a biopsy is commonly used in cases of chronic hepatitis, rather than acute cases of the disease. The test is much like getting a shot, but instead of injecting something, the needle is used to remove a tiny bit of liver. The tissue is then examined under a microscope. Looking at the liver tissue directly allows the doctor to see how much scar tissue and inflammation there are in the liver of a person who has chronic hepatitis. It can also reveal whether cirrhosis is occurring, something otherwise very difficult to detect in its early stages. Doing a liver biopsy also allows doctors to directly test certain minerals and enzymes in the liver tissue, as well as to check for cancer cells.

TREATING HEPATITIS B

The treatment for hepatitis B depends on whether you have the acute or chronic form of the disease. Since hepatitis B is caused by a virus, the treatment for acute hepatitis B is aimed at allowing your body to fight the virus with its own immune system. You will most likely feel tired, so you should get lots of rest and try not to overdo activities. You should avoid alcohol and other drugs, which damage liver cells. As with many viruses, hepatitis B will often clear up without medical treatment. This happens because the cells in your immune system eventually kill the virus. In about 2 percent of people who get hepatitis B, however, the disease causes liver failure.

In about 5 percent of patients, the hepatitis B is not completely killed by the immune system. In these cases, the hepatitis virus remains active, without causing liver failure.

Another 5 to 10 percent of people infected with hepatitis B will not get sick. These people are called hepatitis B carriers. Carriers may not even be aware that they are infected with hepatitis B, so they can easily pass the virus on to other people through their blood, semen, and other bodily fluids. The only ways to protect yourself against infection by carriers is to practice safe sex and get immunized against the hepatitis B virus.

PRESENT MEDICATIONS AND THERAPIES

In the past, there weren't too many options available to those suffering from chronic hepatitis B. However, in recent years several treatments have been developed for the disease. Many of these treatments were developed using genetic engineering techniques. Genetic engineering is the process of changing the genetic material in cells. Gene-based therapies are aimed at reducing the hepatitis B virus (HBV) present in the liver, thus reducing the amount of liver damage.

How do gene-based therapies work? The hepatitis B virus consists of an outer protective shell with a core of deoxyribonucleic acid (DNA). The DNA carries the virus's genetic blueprint. The HBV attaches to the membrane surrounding a cell and injects its DNA into the cell.

The virus's DNA consists of two twisted strands. Each strand is made up of four bases: adenine (A), thymine (T), cytosine (C), and guanine (G). Each type of base in one strand of DNA binds (attaches to) a certain base on the other DNA strand. A binds to T, and C binds to G. This produces a pair of twisted DNA strands attached to each other. Each pair of attached bases is called a base pair.

The current treatments for chronic hepatitis B generally do one of two things: they block the production of a chemical necessary for the reproduction of the virus's DNA, or they insert an inactive form of one of the base pairs used to make the virus's DNA so that it will not work right. Current treatments include:

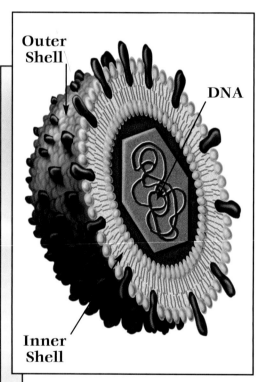

Outer Shell

DNA

Inner Shell

Above is a cutaway view of a hepatitis B virus. The DNA in the virus's central core is copied to make more hepatitis B viruses.

- **Adefovir and Lamivudine.** Adefovir is marketed under the brand names Preveon and Hepasera. It was originally developed by Gilead Sciences to control the HIV virus, which is responsible for AIDS. In 2002, the U.S. Food and Drug Administration (FDA) approved adefovir for the treatment of chronic hepatitis B. Lamivudine is sold under the brand names Zeffix and Epivir. Both adefovir and lamivudine work in a similar fashion: they keep the virus from reproducing by blocking an enzyme in cells that the HBV needs to copy its DNA.

- **Entecavir.** Marketed under the brand name Baraclude, entecavir is an analogue, or substitute, for guanine, one of the bases that make up DNA. Entecavir blocks three steps in the virus's reproduction to reduce the amount of virus in the person's system.
- **Interferon.** Interferons are substances that are naturally produced in the body. They attach to the surface of cells and stimulate the body to put out chemicals that cause various changes. Two types of interferon are used to treat chronic hepatitis B. In the body, interferon attaches itself to the surface of the infected cell. This causes the cell to produce chemicals that keep the HBV from reproducing, and it stimulates the body's immune system cells to attack the HBV.
- **Telbivudine.** Telbivudine is marketed by the pharmaceutical company Novartis under the name Tyzeka. Telbivudine replaces one of the basic elements that make up DNA, preventing the formation of one of the two strands of DNA in the virus.

Unfortunately, these treatments do not always kill the hepatitis B virus. Frequently, they simply keep the virus in check without eliminating it completely. In many cases, a person with chronic hepatitis B must continue to use the treatment indefinitely to keep the virus from starting to reproduce again. In addition, these medications—interferons especially—often cause undesirable side effects, such as fatigue and flu-like symptoms.

Often, chronic hepatitis is treated with a combination of therapies. Attacking the virus with multiple methods is effective because if one approach doesn't work, or if the virus becomes immune to a certain medication, one of the other medicines will often work.

THE SEARCH FOR A CURE

Ideally, scientists would like to be able to cure hepatitis B, rather than just contain it. Many researchers are currently investigating ways to do this. Once again, genetic engineering appears to hold the key to developing a cure. In one project, a group of researchers led by Dr. Gary Clawson at Penn State College of Medicine in Hershey, Pennsylvania, have come up with a way to destroy the DNA of the hepatitis B virus. Their approach has worked successfully in infected mice. They use ribozymes—elements found in the nucleus of cells—to cut up strands of ribonucleic acid (RNA). RNA plays an important role in copying the virus's DNA.

Clawson and his colleagues came up with a way to package ribozymes in a fatty capsule called a liposome.

Extreme Surgery: Liver Transplants

If a person's liver fails completely, the only treatment option is to replace the entire liver with one that functions. This is called a liver transplant. In this procedure, the diseased liver is removed from the patient and a new liver from a recently deceased donor is attached in its place. The patient must then take medication that keeps his or her immune system from rejecting the new liver.

Today, 85 to 90 percent of patients receiving liver transplants survive at least one year, and 65 percent survive at least five years. However, there are two problems with liver transplantation. First, there are not enough livers from donors for all the people who need one. Second, in order for a person's immune system to accept the new liver, it must closely match the blood type and tissue type of the person receiving it. It is not always possible to find suitable livers in a timely manner, so researchers are exploring other ideas. One approach involves "living donor" transplants. For this, a piece of liver is removed from a living person and implanted. The idea is that because of the liver's unique ability to regenerate, it will grow into a full liver. Another approach also relies on the liver's ability to regenerate. In this case, however, researchers use techniques such as implanting liver cells onto a structure made of biodegradable material in a laboratory. The goal is to get them to reproduce, ultimately growing a new liver that can then be transplanted.

They genetically engineered the liposome to seek out liver cells infected with HBV. Once there, the liposome breaks up, releasing the ribozymes. The ribozymes slice up the hepatitis B RNA, making it impossible for the hepatitis B virus to make more copies of its DNA.

Other approaches being explored include inserting inactive artificial hepatitis B DNA into infected cells. This

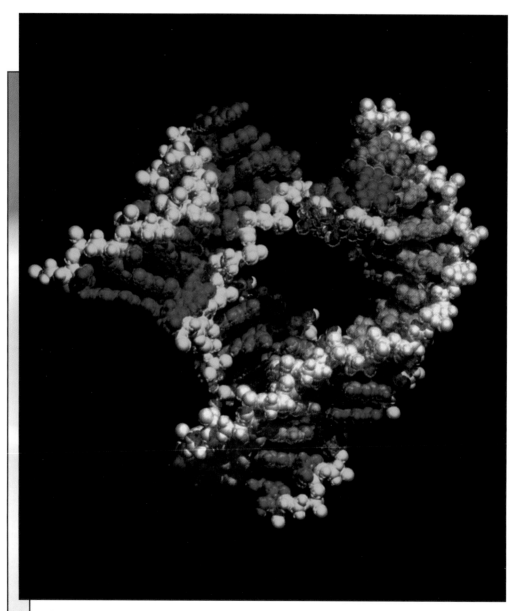

This computer-generated model shows the molecular structure of a ribozyme. Advanced genetic research uses ribozymes to keep hepatitis viruses from reproducing.

artificial hepatitis DNA binds to RNA in place of the real hepatitis DNA, keeping the real hepatitis B virus from making copies of itself. Scientists deliver the DNA to the cells by using plasmids, which are small rings of DNA obtained from bacteria or yeast. Scientists replace a segment of the plasmid DNA with the piece of DNA they want to insert into a cell. They then infect the cell with the plasmids. The new DNA is incorporated into the DNA being produced in the cell. In this case, the idea is to incorporate the artificial piece of DNA into the hepatitis B virus DNA, making it inactive. Early experiments in batches of cells grown in the laboratory and in animals have shown promise. However, it remains to be seen if the plasmids can target liver cells specifically and deliver enough of the artificial DNA.

Yet another approach under investigation is to try to deliver substances (such as proteins) to the liver cells that would keep the virus's outer shell from forming correctly. This approach has also shown promise in both animal models and in cell cultures.

Ten Great Questions to Ask Your Doctor

1. What should I do to optimize my chances of getting better?

2. Is it possible that I have passed on hepatitis B to people I have come into casual contact with?

3. Do the people I live with need to be tested for hepatitis B?

4. Can I participate in sports while I'm infected with hepatitis B?

5. How long will it take to get better?

6. When should I return for a checkup?

7. What should I do if my symptoms don't improve?

8. What are the side effects of the treatment you recommend?

9. How will I recognize if the treatment is working?

10. How will I know when the disease has cleared up?

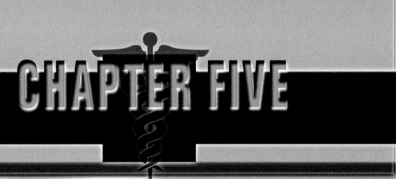

CHAPTER FIVE

Coping with Chronic Hepatitis B

U ntil a cure is found, many people are faced with living with the chronic form of hepatitis B. This chapter looks at the issues related to living with this disease. Two major aspects of living with chronic hepatitis B are the need to treat and protect the liver and the need to protect others from catching the disease.

PROTECTING YOUR HEALTH

If you have hepatitis B, your main concern is taking care of your own health. It is important to keep your body in good shape so that your immune system will do the best job possible of fighting the virus. This means eating a healthy, well-balanced diet. You also need to get enough sleep. Doing these things improves your body's strength and energy. Don't smoke. Smoking damages not only the liver but also many other organs in the body, making your body less able to fight infection.

Since the virus is already damaging cells in your liver, you need to be careful not to consume things that further damage liver cells. You should not drink alcohol or use recreational drugs. These can damage liver cells and break down into toxic chemicals that build up in your body because your damaged liver is not capable of clearing them out. It's not only illegal drugs that you need to be careful with. You need to be careful that you don't take prescription or over-the-counter medications that can hurt your liver. Before you take new over-the-counter

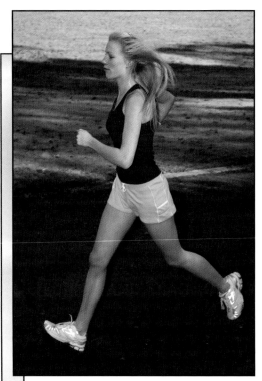

Staying in good shape by exercising is crucial. Physical strength makes your body better able to deal with the effects of chronic hepatitis.

medicine, check with the pharmacist to find out if there are any problems with taking it when you have liver disease. Likewise, make sure that any doctor you see knows that you have hepatitis B. The doctor will need to check that any medication prescribed won't affect your liver. Your doctor may also need to adjust the dose because your liver will not remove it from your bloodstream as fast as a healthy liver would. Do not use herbal supplements without checking

Resources for Coping with Hepatitis

Coping with hepatitis B, especially the chronic type, can be stressful. You have to deal with the disease itself and the social aspects of dealing with others who may not understand the disease.

There are several sources of support for people with hepatitis B. One is friends and family. Another is professionals such as psychiatrists, psychologists, and counselors. These professionals are trained to help individuals cope with trauma and stress. They are particularly useful if having hepatitis B leads to psychological disorders such as depression (an excessive feeling of sadness).

A third source of help is support groups. These are made up of other people who suffer from hepatitis B. Because they have the same problem, they can understand what you are going through. People in support groups provide emotional support to each other. In addition, they share useful tips and information in areas such as new treatments. There are two types of support groups: in-person groups and online groups. Your doctor or local hospital may be able to provide information on support groups that meet in your area. In addition, many of the organizations listed in the back of this book provide information on support groups.

Online support groups consist of people who share information and advice over the Internet. One such support group is the Hepatitis B Information and Support Group (http://www.hblist.org), which includes people from all over the world. Major search engine sites such as Google and Yahoo! Groups often include informal support groups for people with diseases, including hepatitis B. However, when dealing with information you receive from people over the Internet, remember that it is just like talking to people in person. Their information is based on personal opinion and experience. So, before taking any action based on it, be sure to check with your doctor.

with your doctor. These plants get their effects from the chemicals they contain, just like manufactured medicines. Your doctor can tell you if a specific supplement is safe for you to use.

In order to stay as healthy as you can and catch any issues as soon as possible, you should see your doctor regularly for checkups—at least once or twice a year. This allows the doctor to notice any changes in your condition and treat them rapidly.

PROTECTING OTHERS

It is important to understand that when you have hepatitis B, you can spread it to other people who live with you, even if you do not have sex with them. This includes other family members. When the virus is in your blood, you can pass it along to another person if that person comes in contact with your blood. This might happen, for instance, if you cut yourself and someone in your house picks up a towel that you used to wrap around the wound. If others have cuts or scratches that allow the virus through their skin, they can catch the disease. Anything that might have your blood on it such as a razor, nail scissors, or toothbrush could have the virus on it. For this reason, anyone you live with should be tested for the virus and vaccinated for protection. Be aware, however, that the virus isn't spread by casual contact such as hugging, so you do not need to refrain from contact with other people.

If you develop a relationship with someone, you need to tell that person that you have hepatitis. If you don't feel comfortable talking to him or her, you shouldn't be having sex with that person. He or she should be vaccinated before you have sex. If you are a female who has hepatitis and someday you get pregnant, within twelve hours of birth your baby will need to get a shot of a special hepatitis B antibody called hepatitis B immunoglobulin. This antigen provides short-term protection for the baby until further treatment can be given. Your baby should also receive a

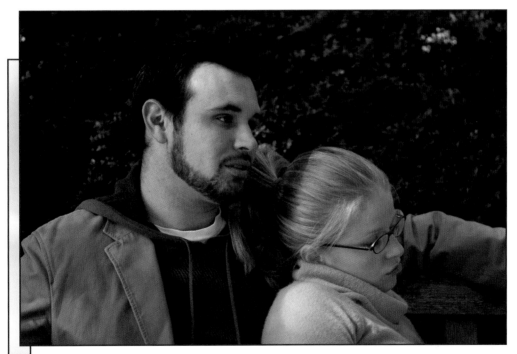

Communication is an important part of a healthy relationship. You need to be able to discuss serious issues—such as the fact that you have hepatitis B.

full course (usually three shots over a six-month period) of the regular hepatitis B vaccination.

Above all, it's important to maintain as normal a lifestyle as possible and maintain healthy relationships. When they take care of themselves, most people with hepatitis B live long, productive lives.

GLOSSARY

aborigine Person native to a region.

acute Short-term but severe. Applies to diseases in which a patient is sick for a short time.

analogue Something that is similar to a naturally occurring element in the body.

antibody Protein that attaches to foreign particles in the body so that other immune system cells can recognize and destroy those particles.

antigen Substance that sets off an immune system reaction and causes the formation of antibodies.

atom Smallest building block of an element, such as hydrogen.

bile Liquid produced in the liver that breaks down fat.

cholesterol Fatty substance from which some hormones are made.

cirrhosis Forming of scar tissue in the liver.

clot In terms of blood, to coagulate or stop flowing freely.

contagious Able to spread from person to person.

deceased Dead.

DNA (deoxyribonucleic acid) Material that encodes our genetic information.

enzyme Protein in the body that must be present for certain reactions to take place.

epidemic Rapid spread of a disease to a large number of people.

gland Organ that produces a chemical that affects the body.

hepatocyte Liver cell.

hormone Chemical that controls a body process.

immune system Body system that protects against dangerous foreign organisms and substances.

indefinitely Having no set ending time.

inflammation Swelling, pain, and heat in a tissue or organ.

jaundice Yellowing of the skin and whites of the eyes caused by a diseased liver.

lobe Rounded segment of an organ.

membrane Thin layer of tissue that covers an organ.

optimize Maximize; make as good as possible.

pore Small opening through which fluid can pass.

regenerate Grow back.

RNA (ribonucleic acid) Material in cells that plays a key role in making copies of DNA.

secrete Produce a fluid in body cells or organs.

serum Clear, watery part of blood in which blood cells float.

sieve Strainer or device used to refine a substance.

stroke Blocking of a blood vessel in the brain, often caused by a blood clot.

toxin Poison.

FOR MORE INFORMATION

American Association for the Study of Liver Diseases
1001 North Fairfax, Suite 400
Alexandria, VA 22314
(703) 299-9766
Web site: https://www.aasld.org
This organization for liver disease researchers provides
publications, and its Web site has a "Patient
Resources" section with a physician referral list, and
information on hepatitis screening, liver transplants,
and liver disease, as well as health tips.

American Liver Foundation
75 Malden Lane, Suite 603
New York, NY 10038
(212) 668-1000
Web site: http://www.liverfoundation.org
This organization provides a variety of resources, including
brochures and Webcasts, related to liver disease for
patients, friends, and families. It has local chapters
throughout the United States.

American Social Health Association
P.O. Box 13827

Research Triangle Park, NC 27709

(919) 361-8400

(800) 227-8922 (STD Resource Center Hotline)

Web site: http://www.ashastd.org/index.cfm

This site provides information on hepatitis B and general
information on safe sex.

Canadian Liver Foundation

Suite 1500-2235 Sheppard Avenue East

Toronto, ON M2J 5B5

Canada

(416) 491-3353

(800) 563-5483

Web site: http://www.liver.ca

This organization provides a wide range of information
and patient support resources.

Hepatitis B Foundation

3805 Old Easton Road

Doylestown, PA 18902

(215) 489-4900

Web site: http://www.hepb.org

This organization provides the latest news on hepatitis B
and a variety of resources, including publications.

Hepatitis Foundation International

504 Blick Drive

Silver Spring, MD 20904

(800) 891-0707

Web site: http://www.hepfi.org

This organization provides a wide variety of information on living with hepatitis, a list of support groups, helpful booklets, and news.

WEB SITES

Due to the changing nature of Internet links, Rosen Publishing has developed an online list of Web sites related to the subject of this book. This site is updated regularly. Please use this link to access the list:

http://www.rosenlinks.com/lsh/hepa

FOR FURTHER READING

Booley, Theresa Anne. *Alcohol and Your Liver: The Incredibly Disgusting Story*. New York, NY: Rosen Publishing Group, Inc., 2000.

Everson, Gregory T., Hedy Weinberg, and Steve Bingham. *Living with Hepatitis B: A Survivor's Guide*. Long Island City, NY: Hatherleigh Press, 2001.

Geddes, Louise, ed. *Contemporary Issues Companion: Sexually Transmitted Diseases*. Chicago, IL: Greenhaven Press, 2002.

Green, William Finley. *The First Year—Hepatitis B: An Essential Guide for the Newly Diagnosed*. Cambridge, MA: Marlowe and Co., 2002.

Hatchell, Deborah. *What Smart Teenagers Know . . . About Dating, Relationships, & Sex*. Ventura, CA: Piper Books, 2003.

Holmes, Melissa, and Trish Hutchison. *Girlology Hang-Ups, Hook-Ups, and Holding Out: Stuff You Need to Know About Your Body, Sex, & Dating*. New York, NY: Chelsea House, 2007.

Hunter, Miranda, and William Hunter. *Staying Safe: A Teen's Guide to Sexually Transmitted Diseases*. Broomall, PA: Mason Crest, 2004.

Kdesnikow, Tassia. *Diseases and Disorders: Sexually Transmitted Diseases.* San Diego, CA: Lucent Books, 2003.

Radzsizewicz, Tina. *Ready or Not? A Girl's Guide to Making Her Own Decisions About Dating, Love, and Sex.* New York, NY: Walker, 2006.

Stanley, Deborah. *Sexual Health Information for Teens: Health Tips About Sexual Development, Human Reproduction, and Sexually Transmitted Diseases.* Detroit, MI: Omnigraphics, 2003.

BIBLIOGRAPHY

Guttmacher Institute. "Facts on American Teens' Sexual and Reproductive Health." September 2006. Retrieved January 18, 2008 (http://www.guttmacher.org/pubs/fb_ATSRH.html).

Karayiannis, Peter. "Hepatitis B Virus: Old, New, and Future Approaches to Antiviral Treatment." *Journal of Antimicrobial Chemotherapy*, Vol. 51, March 13, 2003. Retrieved January 19, 2008 (http://jac.oxfordjournals.org/cgi/content/full/51/4/761).

MayoClinic.com. "Hepatitis B." Retrieved January 12, 2008 (http://www.mayoclinic.com/health/hepatitis-b/DS00398/DSECTION=2).

Palmer, Melissa. *Hepatitis and Liver Disease*. New York, NY: Penguin, 2004.

Patrick, David M., et al. "Elimination of Acute Hepatitis B Among Adolescents After One Decade of an Immunization Program Targeting Grade 6 Students." *Pediatric Infectious Disease Journal*, January 12, 2003. Retrieved January 19, 2008 (http://www.medscape.com/viewarticle/463130).

Pharmaceutical News. "Tiny Ribozyme Package Could Be Future Treatment of Hepatitis B Virus." March 22,

2004. Retrieved January 19, 2008 (http://www.news-medical.net/?id=93).

Tran, Tram T. "AASLD 2006—Clinical Advances in Hepatitis B and Hepatitis C." American Association for the Study of Liver Diseases. Retrieved January 12, 2008 (http://www.medscape.com/viewarticle/548122).

World Health Organization. "Hepatitis B." October 2000. Retrieved January 12, 2008 (http://www.who.int/mediacentre/factsheets/fs204/en).

Worman, Howard J. *The Liver Disorders and Hepatitis Sourcebook*. New York, NY: McGraw-Hill, 2006.

INDEX

ABOUT THE AUTHOR

Jeri Freedman has a B.A. degree from Harvard University. For fifteen years, Freedman worked for companies in the medical field. She is the author of twenty-five young adult nonfiction books, many published by Rosen Publishing. Among her previous titles are Hemophilia; Lymphoma: Current and Emerging Trends in Detection and Treatment; How Do We Know About Genetics and Heredity?; The Mental and Physical Effects of Obesity; and Autism.

PHOTO CREDITS

Cover © www.istockphoto.com/Chris Schmidt; pp. 1, 15 CDC; p. 4 © www.istockphoto.com/ericsphotography; p. 4 (silhouette) © www.istockphoto.com/jamesbenet; pp. 5, 11 © Superstock, Inc.; p. 8 © Nucleus Medical Art/Visuals Unlimited; pp. 17, 26, 48 Shutterstock.com; p. 19 CDC/Dr. Thomas F. Sellers/Emory University; p. 21 Chris Anderson/Aurora/Getty Images; p. 31 dpa/Newscom; p. 33 Paul Burns/Blend Images/Getty Images; p. 37 Khaled Desouki/AFP/Getty Images; p. 40 © Mark Miller/Photo Researchers, Inc.; p. 44 © Kenneth Eward/Photo Researchers, Inc.; p. 51 © www.istockphoto.com/Timothy Babasade; back cover (top to bottom) 3D4Medical.com/Getty Images, © www.istockphoto.com/Luis Carlos Torres, © www.istockphoto.com/Kiyoshi Takahase Segundo, CDC, © www.istockphoto.com/Amanda Rohde, Scott Bodell/Photodisc/Getty Images.

Designer: Nelson Sá; **Editor:** Christopher Roberts
Photo Researcher: Cindy Reiman